LEARNER ACTIVITIES WORKBOOK FOR

# Core Competencies of Civility

## in nursing & healthcare

Cynthia Clark, PhD, RN, ANEF, FAAN
Jessica G. Smith, PhD, RN

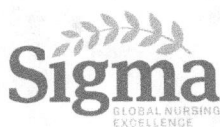

**Sigma**
GLOBAL NURSING
EXCELLENCE

*Sigma Theta Tau International Honor Society of Nursing (Sigma) is a nonprofit organization whose mission is developing nurse leaders anywhere to improve healthcare everywhere. Founded in 1922, Sigma has more than 135,000 active members in over 100 countries and territories. Members include practicing nurses, instructors, researchers, policymakers, entrepreneurs, and others. Sigma's more than 540 chapters are located at more than 700 institutions of higher education throughout Armenia, Australia, Botswana, Brazil, Canada, Colombia, Croatia, England, Eswatini, Ghana, Hong Kong, Ireland, Israel, Italy, Jamaica, Japan, Jordan, Kenya, Lebanon, Malawi, Mexico, the Netherlands, Nigeria, Pakistan, Philippines, Portugal, Puerto Rico, Scotland, Singapore, South Africa, South Korea, Sweden, Taiwan, Tanzania, Thailand, the United States, and Wales. Learn more at www.sigmanursing.org.*

Sigma Theta Tau International
550 West North Street
Indianapolis, IN, USA 46202

To request a review copy for course adoption, order additional books, buy in bulk, or purchase for corporate use, contact Sigma Marketplace at 888.654.4968 (US/Canada toll-free), +1.317.687.2256 (International), or solutions@sigmamarketplace.org.

To request author information, or for speaker or other media requests, contact Sigma Marketing at 888.634.7575 (US/Canada toll-free) or +1.317.634.8171 (International).

ISBN:       9781646480722
PDF ISBN: 9781646480739

First Printing, 2022

**Publisher:** Dustin Sullivan                    **Managing Editor:** Carla Hall
**Acquisitions Editor:** Emily Hatch              **Publications Specialist:** Todd Lothery
**Development Editor:** Jill Stanley              **Project Editor:** Alexandra Andrzejewski
**Cover Designer:** Rebecca Batchelor            **Copy Editor:** Todd Lothery
**Interior Design/Page Layout:** Rebecca Batchelor  **Proofreader:** Todd Lothery

# About the Authors

**Cynthia Clark, PhD, RN, ANEF, FAAN,** is founder of *Civility Matters* and Professor Emeritus at Boise State University. As a clinician, she specialized in adolescent mental health, substance abuse intervention and recovery, and suicide and violence prevention. She is a leading expert in fostering civility and healthy work environments around the globe. Her groundbreaking work on fostering civility has brought national and international attention to the controversial issues of incivility in academic and work environments. Her theory-driven interventions, empirical measurements, theoretical models, and reflective assessments provide best practices to prevent, measure, and address uncivil behavior and to create healthy workplaces.

**Jessica G. Smith, PhD, RN,** is an Assistant Professor at the University of Texas at Arlington College of Nursing and Health Innovation. She received her PhD in nursing from the University of Wisconsin-Milwaukee in 2016. She completed a two-year postdoctoral fellowship (2016–2018) at the Center for Health Outcomes and Policy Research at the University of Pennsylvania. Her areas of interest include understanding the needs of the acute rural nurse workforce to deliver safer patient care and how work environments and processes influence nurse well-being.

# Table of Contents

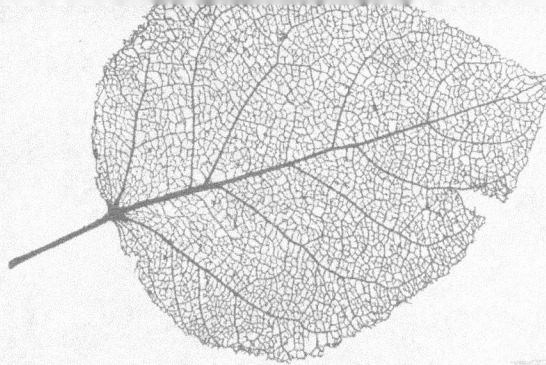

# 1

# What Is Civility, and Why Does It Matter?

# Key Concepts

After reading the chapter, test your understanding of the concepts with short answers.

1. What is civility?

_____

_____

_____

_____

2. Describe the difference between being "merely" civil and "authentically" civil. Then, explain the outcomes of authentic civility.

_____

_____

_____

_____

3. Discuss how interacting with civility is a choice.

_____

_____

_____

_____

4. Describe the ethical imperative for civility.

_____

_____

_____

_____

5. What are the concepts of the Conceptual Model for Achieving a Culture of Belonging?

_____

_____

_____

_____

6. How do the concepts of the Conceptual Model for Achieving a Culture of Belonging interrelate?

_____

_____

_____

_____

7. What are the definitions of diversity, equity, and inclusion?

_____

_____

_____

_____

# Rationale for Implementation

After reading the chapter, test your understanding of the concepts with short answers.

1. Why does civility matter in work and learning environments?

_____

_____

_____

_____

2. Why is it important for an organization to foster a culture of belonging?

_____

_____

_____

_____

## Application of the Concepts

Working with a small group, complete the following exercise as directed by your facilitator(s).

### 1. Group Activity: Understanding the Conceptual Model for Achieving a Culture of Belonging

Imagine that you are a member of a team of nurses or a nursing faculty group charged with improving the culture of your work or learning environment. Working in teams of five to six members, describe your basic understanding of how the Conceptual Model for Achieving a Culture of Belonging might be used to frame the process.

_____

_____

_____

_____

## Reflection

Reflection is an integral aspect of learning, involving inquiry, discussion, and problem-solving. In this section, reflect on what you have learned from Chapter 1 by sharing ideas, takeaways, application of information, and thoughtful feedback. Working in small groups, teams, or learning circles is a learner-centered approach designed to inspire collaboration and build synergy by problem-solving together.

1. Think about what civility meant to you before you read this chapter compared to after. Was there anything you learned about civility that you did not consider before? Why or why not? Going forward, how do you see yourself as a member of the healthcare professions fostering a culture of belonging?

_____

_____

_____

_____

2. Using the Civility Reflection provided in Chapter 1, describe how your life events and experiences have impacted your worldview, your life, and the lives of others.

_____

_____

_____

_____

Take a moment to sit in silence and reflect. If you wish, record your thoughts in a journal. Think deeply and introspectively about your childhood and adolescence. Where and when does your story begin? Where did you grow up and go to school? Did you travel to far-off places or stay mainly in your backyard? How have your life events and experiences shaped the person you have become and continue to become? How have these events and experiences impacted your life and the lives of others around you? Who were the most influential people of your childhood? What lessons did you learn? How are the lessons still affecting your life today? If you are inclined, share your story with a trusted friend, family member, or colleague.

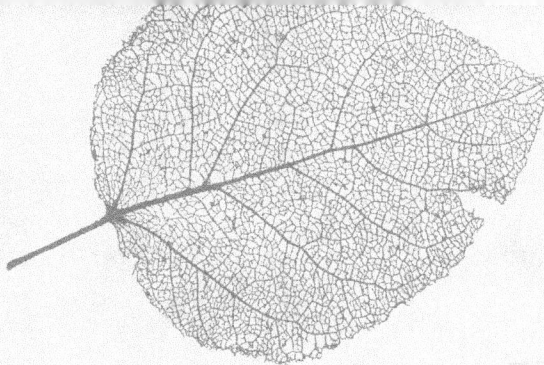

# 2

# The Detrimental Impact of Workplace Aggression

## LEARNING OUTCOMES

- Describe the impact of workplace aggression in healthcare for patients, healthcare workers, nursing educators, nursing students, and new nurses.

- Using the Continuum of Workplace Aggression, describe the impact of unaddressed lower-level forms of aggression that can occur in the workplace.

- Define the different forms of workplace violence according to the National Institute for Occupational Safety & Health.

- Identify barriers to addressing workplace aggression.

# Key Concepts

After reading the chapter, test your understanding of the concepts with short answers.

- What are potential risks of experiencing incivility in the workplace for patients?

_____

_____

_____

_____

- What are potential risks of workplace aggression for healthcare workers?

_____

_____

_____

_____

- What are potential risks of workplace aggression for nursing educators and students?

_____

_____

_____

_____

- What is the potential impact of workplace aggression on a new nurse's well-being?

_____

_____

_____

_____

- What is the Continuum of Workplace Aggression?

  _____

  _____

  _____

  _____

- What are the National Institute for Occupational Safety & Health (NIOSH) definitions of violence?

  _____

  _____

  _____

  _____

- Why don't nurses report workplace aggression?

  _____

  _____

  _____

  _____

# Rationale for Implementation

After reading the chapter, test your understanding of the concepts with short answers.

1. Why is it important for nurses, healthcare providers, and educators to identify and understand the impact of workplace aggression?

   _____

   _____

   _____

   _____

2. Why is it important to report workplace aggression?

_____

_____

_____

_____

# Application of the Concepts

Working with a partner and individually, complete the following exercises as directed by your facilitator(s).

## 1. Paired Activity: Sharing an Uncivil Encounter

Recall an uncivil encounter you had in the past in nursing, healthcare, or the education setting. Think about the events preceding it, the event, and the aftermath. Then, share this experience and reflections about it in a conversation with a trusted friend or colleague. Ask your colleague to share their thoughts on the following questions regarding the event.

1. Have you ever experienced something like this?

_____

_____

_____

_____

2. How would you feel if you experienced this situation?

_____

_____

_____

_____

3. If faced with this situation, what would you do? Explain your reasoning.

_____

_____

_____

_____

Once finished, you may switch with your friend or colleague and ask them to share their experience, and you can share your responses to the same set of questions.

Share your biggest takeaways from your discussions with the larger group.

## 2. Case Narrative Activity: Bystander of an Uncivil Shift Report

Read the following narrative, reflect on the content and impact of the situation, and respond to the questions that follow by taking notes.

### Narrative: The Case of the Bystander of an Uncivil Shift Report

Lindsey, a staff registered nurse, enters a busy oncology unit at the beginning of her shift and witnesses a heated, uncivil exchange from an oncoming nurse who is already receiving report from an off-going nurse. The situation is about tasks left undone, and the oncoming nurse is angry and talking down to the nurse who was giving report and soon to be off shift: "You've got to be kidding me. Really? What have you done all shift? Why can't you manage your time better? I'm sick and tired of cleaning up after you!" The off-going nurse appears intimidated and shocked at what is happening.

As directed by your facilitator, take some time to answer the following questions, taking notes so you can remember your answers. Then pair up with a partner and share your answers. Finally, choose one takeaway that the pair of you found most insightful and share that with the class.

**Questions:**

1. If you were the third-party nurse witnessing the event, how would you feel?

_____

_____

_____

_____

2. What would you do or not do, and why?

_____

_____

_____

_____

3. How might this situation impact the clinical setting and patient care?

_____

_____

_____

_____

4. What are some barriers to addressing the situation?

_____

_____

_____

_____

5. What measures might you take to overcome these barriers?

_____

_____

_____

_____

# Reflection

The process of reflection helps you become more self-aware, problem-solve, and identify motivators and barriers that may impact how you recognize and address challenging situations. You can engage in reflective practice through dialogue in small and large groups or writing activities such as journaling, free-writing, scriptwriting, or narrative storytelling. Use the following reflective questions to apply the concepts from this chapter.

1. Did your perspective about the impact of workplace aggression change after reading this chapter? Why or why not? If it did change, describe what you learned and how it informs your future practice.

   _____

   _____

   _____

   _____

2. Let's say you witnessed low-level uncivil behavior in the workplace since having read this chapter. What are the potential implications of leaving this behavior unaddressed? How motivated would you be to address uncivil behavior, knowing the impact it can have on patient safety? What would be a barrier to addressing uncivil behavior as a witness, and how could you overcome this barrier?

   _____

   _____

   _____

   _____

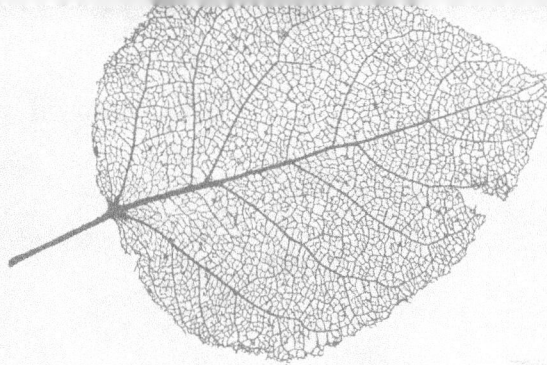

# 3

# The Power and Imperative of Self-Awareness

### LEARNING OUTCOMES

- Define emotional intelligence and its relationship to self-awareness.

- Explain the importance of self-awareness for fostering civil relationships.

- Describe at least two strategies to improve self-awareness.

- Discuss how explicit and implicit biases might contribute to incivility.

- Utilize the IAT from Project Implicit to increase self-awareness about potential implicit biases.

## Key Concepts

After reading the chapter, test your understanding of the concepts with short answers.

• How would you define emotional intelligence?

_____

_____

_____

_____

• What is the relationship between emotional intelligence and self-awareness?

_____

_____

_____

_____

• Identify at least two strategies to improve self-awareness.

_____

_____

_____

_____

• Define explicit and implicit bias.

_____

_____

_____

_____

• How do explicit and implicit biases relate to incivility?

_____

_____

_____

_____

## Rationale for Implementation

After reading the chapter, test your understanding of the concepts with short answers.

1. Why is improving self-awareness important to fostering civil relationships?

_____

_____

_____

_____

2. Why is it important to acknowledge explicit and implicit biases in relation to civility in nursing and healthcare?

_____

_____

_____

_____

# Application of the Concepts

Working with a small group and partner, complete the following exercises as directed by your facilitator(s).

## 1. Group Activity: Using the Implicit Association Test to Build Self-Awareness

Complete at least one of the Implicit Association Tests (IAT) provided by Project Implicit (https://implicit.harvard.edu/implicit/).

Using the following questions, share your insights with a small group, as directed by your facilitator(s):

1. Which IAT did you complete? What factors motivated you to select this test?

_____

_____

_____

_____

2. Using only one word, how would you describe the IAT experience?

_____

_____

_____

_____

3. Which results or findings from the IAT surprised you the most?

_____

_____

_____

_____

4. Which results or findings from the IAT concerned you the most?

_____

_____

_____

_____

5. What action(s) would you take based on the findings from your IAT?

_____

_____

_____

_____

## 2. Paired Activity: Understand the Impact of Biased Statements

Listed below are examples of biased statements that may be considered uncivil. Read them aloud to your assigned partner, as directed by your facilitator(s), and then answer the following questions.

"Old people are boring."

"This patient is a frequent flyer."

"People from small towns are uneducated."

"Asians are great at math."

"Most male nurses are gay."

"All adolescents are addicted to social media."

"Overweight people are lazy."

Answer the following questions:

1. After reading the examples aloud, what effect did they have on you?

_____

_____

_____

_____

2. Have you been on the receiving end, or observed, biased statements?

_____

_____

_____

_____

3. How did experiencing or witnessing biased statements impact you?

_____

_____

_____

_____

4. If you have witnessed or experienced statements like these in the workplace, how did you respond or not respond?

_____

_____

_____

_____

5. If you chose to respond, what was the outcome?

_____

_____

_____

_____

6. If you chose not to respond, what was the outcome?

_____

_____

_____

_____

7. What might you do differently in the future?

_____

_____

_____

_____

As directed by your facilitator(s), be prepared to share your responses with your classmates.

# Reflection

The process of reflection helps you become more self-aware, introspective, and mindful of the impact your behaviors have on others and the work environment. Reflective activities provide an opportunity for inquiry and a mechanism for questioning ideas, assumptions, and beliefs. When you share your insights and perspectives with others, it provides an opportunity to receive feedback and additional points of view from other individuals.

For this reflection exercise, you can choose to complete the Workplace Civility Index or the Everyday Civility Index provided in Chapter 3.

To complete the index of choice, find a quiet place, free from distractions, and honestly assess your level of civility. Then, respond to the following questions:

1. How satisfied are you with your overall civility score?

_____

_____

_____

_____

2. Are there examples of civility where you excel?

_____

_____

_____

_____

3. Are there examples of civility you wish to improve?

_____

_____

_____

_____

4. In the most honest way possible, determine one or more areas for civility improvement and personal growth. Then identify one or more strategies you will implement to improve an area of civility and personal growth. Include your proposed timeline for implementation.

_____

_____

_____

_____

5. In the most honest way possible, identify one or more areas of strength. Then identify one or more strategies you will implement to continue developing these strengths. Include your proposed timeline for implementation.

_____

_____

_____

_____

Once you have completed your index of choice and responded to these questions, your facilitator(s) may ask you to select a classmate, colleague, or friend and take turns sharing your insights and reflections.

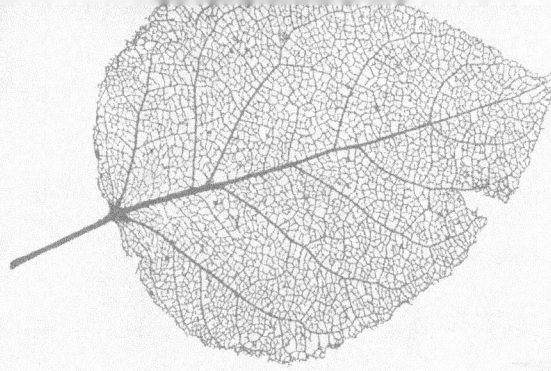

# 4

# Practicing the Fundamentals of Civility

## LEARNING OUTCOMES

- Define and describe what it means to be a civilist.

- Explain how expressing gratitude is a fundamental element of civility.

- Describe how living by the Platinum Rule is a fundamental element of civility.

- Define how conveying empathy is a fundamental element of civility.

- Explain how listening well is a fundamental element of civility.

- Describe how expressing microaffirmations is a fundamental element of civility.

# Key Concepts

After reading the chapter, test your understanding of the concepts with short answers.

1. Define and describe the characteristics of a civilist.

   _____

   _____

   _____

   _____

2. Define and give an example of each of the five fundamentals of civility.

   - Expressing gratitude means:

   _____

   _____

   _____

   _____

   - Living by the Platinum Rule means:

   _____

   _____

   _____

   _____

   - Conveying empathy means:

   _____

   _____

   _____

   _____

- Listening well means:

  _____

  _____

  _____

  _____

- Expressing micro-affirmations means:

  _____

  _____

  _____

  _____

# Rationale for Implementation

After reading the chapter, test your understanding of the concepts with short answers.

1. Why is it important to strive to be a civilist according to the author's definition?

   _____

   _____

   _____

   _____

2. Why is it important to identify, understand, and practice the fundamentals of civility in nursing and healthcare?

   _____

   _____

   _____

   _____

# Application of the Concepts

Working with a small group and independently, complete the following exercises as directed by your facilitator(s).

## 1. Group Activity: Reflection on What It Means to Be a Civilist

As directed by your facilitator, spend some time thinking about the following questions and developing your definition of a civilist. Then share your responses in a small group.

1. For many learners, the term *civilist* may be a new concept. After reflecting on the author's definition of a civilist, consider how this concept resonates with you in your nursing or healthcare role.

   _____

   _____

   _____

   _____

2. Does the author's characterization align with your definition of a civilist? If not, how might you amend the definition?

   _____

   _____

   _____

   _____

3. As you consider your role in nursing or healthcare:

   • Which aspects of the civilist definition apply to you most?

   _____

   _____

   _____

   _____

- Which aspects of the civilist definition apply to you least?

  _____

  _____

  _____

  _____

- How will you implement the elements of your civilist definition into your nursing or healthcare practice and/or learning environment?

  _____

  _____

  _____

  _____

## 2. Free-Write Activity: Applying the Fundamentals of Civility

Follow these steps to explore one of the fundamentals of civility that most intrigues you.

1. After conducting an internet search on the five fundamentals of civility, select one fundamental that resonates or intrigues you the most.

   _____

   _____

   _____

   _____

2. During a 10-minute free-write, describe how you would integrate this fundamental concept into your work or learning environment.

   _____

   _____

   _____

   _____

To become a civilist, it is important to reflect on behavior that is, and is not, consistent with being a respectful person, and to think about strategies to consistently demonstrate respect. To improve civility acumen, reflect on a time when you or someone you know was treated in a disrespectful or demeaning manner. Then, share your answers to the following questions with a trusted colleague, friend, or family member.

1. Briefly describe the uncivil or disrespectful situation or encounter.

_____

_____

_____

_____

2. As you witnessed or experienced the situation or encounter:

- What feelings were evoked?

_____

_____

_____

_____

- How did you respond to the situation or encounter?

_____

_____

_____

_____

- Were other individuals involved in the situation or encounter? If so, how did they respond?

_____

_____

_____

_____

Now, think of a time when you were affirmed and made to feel valued and respected— your efforts celebrated.

1. Briefly describe the experience of being affirmed and valued by others.

_____

_____

_____

_____

2. As you experienced being affirmed and valued by others:

   • What feelings were evoked?

   _____

   _____

   _____

   • How did you respond to the affirmation?

   _____

   _____

   _____

   • Were there other individuals involved in the experience? If so, how did they respond?

   _____

   _____

   _____

   _____

Reflect on opportunities to integrate micro-affirmations in your everyday work, such as during team meetings or through personal communication. Create a list of micro-affirmations that you can use in your work setting and in everyday encounters.

To help you get started, refer to these examples from page 65 of the book:

- You are absolutely one of the best problem-solvers I know. Thanks!

- You have really opened my eyes and helped me see things in a new light.

- Congratulations on your promotion. It is well deserved.

- Having you on the team has been a game-changer for us.

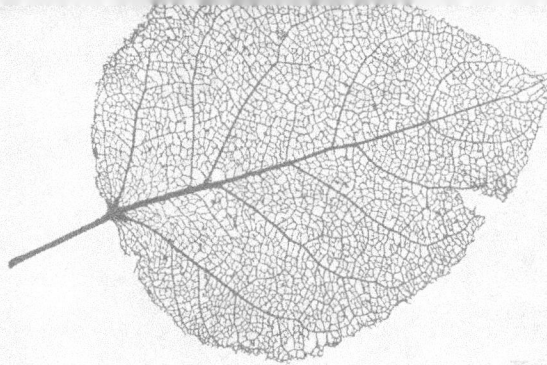

# 5

# Honing Communication Skills and Conflict Competence

## LEARNING OUTCOMES

- Understand the meaning of POWER skills.

- Apply the individual conflict-competence model.

- Employ "I" statements effectively.

- Use learning scripts and phrases to address uncivil or conflicted situations.

- Implement evidence-based frameworks to prevent and address incivility and protect worker and patient safety.

# Key Concepts

After reading the chapter, test your understanding of the concepts with short answers.

1. What does the author mean by POWER skills?

   _____

   _____

   _____

   _____

2. Why are POWER skills challenging to master?

   _____

   _____

   _____

3. Why might it be helpful to think of a situation as a "controversy with civility" rather than as a "conflict?"

   _____

   _____

   _____

   _____

4. Why is it important for nurses, faculty, students, and others to identify their hot buttons and to implement strategies to mitigate the effects of these hot buttons?

   _____

   _____

   _____

   _____

5.   What are the three steps of the individual conflict competence model?

   a. _____

   _____

   _____

   _____

   b. _____

   _____

   _____

   _____

   c. _____

   _____

   _____

   _____

6.   Based on the work of Maxfield and Grenny (2017), describe two common reasons why a nurse might fail to speak up, even though patient safety is at stake.

   a. _____

   _____

   _____

   _____

   b. _____

   _____

   _____

   _____

7.  List the five steps for using "I" statements effectively.

Step 1: _____

Step 2: _____

Step 3: _____

Step 4: _____

Step 5: _____

8.  What are some benefits of using "I" statements when communicating and or attempting to resolve conflict?

_____

_____

_____

_____

9.  List the six steps of the Caring Feedback Model:

Step 1: _____

Step 2: _____

Step 3: _____

Step 4: _____

Step 5: _____

Step 6: _____

10. List the three considerations of the CUS Model:

Step 1: _____

Step 2: _____

Step 3: _____

11.   List the four steps of the DESC Model:

Step 1: _____

Step 2: _____

Step 3: _____

Step 4: _____

12.   List the five steps of the PAAIL Method:

Step 1: _____

Step 2: _____

Step 3: _____

Step 4: _____

Step 5: _____

# Rationale for Implementation

After reading the chapter, test your understanding of the concepts with short answers.

1.   In what ways can strong POWER skills improve patient care, learner engagement, and workplace civility?

_____

_____

_____

_____

2.   What are some characteristics of a good listener? Do you have a good listener in your life? Share an example a colleague, friend, or classmate.

_____

_____

_____

_____

# Application of the Concepts

When teaching this material, the author likes to use a technique called Cognitive Rehearsal (CR), a behavioral strategy whereby groups and individuals work with a skilled facilitator to practice and rehearse effective ways to address uncivil encounters. Facilitators of CR use role-play and simulation to have individuals repeatedly rehearse an uncivil situation, while simultaneously coaching the person to use effective communication and conflict skills and then debriefing the situation. This is a powerful combination of skill sets and is more likely to lead to a successful outcome, improve collaboration and teamwork, and ultimately protect worker and patient safety.

The following activities provide CR scenarios for each of the main conflict resolution models described in Chapter 5. Prior to participating in one or more of these activities, as assigned by the facilitator, read the details of each model carefully, taking notes to make sure you are familiar with the basic concept and steps of each.

Working with a partner and small group, complete the following exercises as directed by your facilitator(s).

## 1. Paired Activity: Using "I" Statements Effectively

With your partner, review the five steps of using "I" statements. Using the following narrative, play the roles and practice using "I" statements to resolve the conflict. Then switch roles and practice them again.

### Narrative: The Case of Intrusive Behavior From a Colleague

Professor Chan is an established, tenured faculty member recently hired at a new university. Professor Chan does not share a lot about herself or about her other teaching and service duties outside of research, but her focus on an established program of research is public. Professor Kelley, a practice and teaching expert colleague and longtime employee of the institution, stops Professor Chan in the hallway of their office and begins to ask pointed and personal questions about her workload and responsibilities. Professor Kelley asked a particularly loaded question, which was, "What do you do with all of your time if you aren't teaching?" Later, Professor Chan overhears Professor Kelley discussing Professor Chan with another colleague in the building, stating, "Everyone here teaches; it's what we are known for in this department. The other faculty work hard teaching the students, going to clinical sites, and grading. Why does Professor Chan get special treatment? What does she even do with research?" Professor Chan is concerned that these messages spreading across the department could result in difficulties collaborating with others and decides it is time to address Professor Kelley's concerns in a meeting. Professor Chan is going to use "I" messaging to frame the discussion.

After your CR of using "I" statements, complete the following reflection questions:

- What was most challenging for you during this role-play exercise?

  _____

  _____

  _____

  _____

- What was most comfortable for you during this role-play exercise?

  _____

  _____

  _____

  _____

## 2. Paired Activity: Caspersen's Framework

Caspersen's Framework is a couple of sentences that you simply fill in to fit the situation. The sentences are: When (the triggering event) happened, I (felt or I believed) ____ because my (need/interest) is important to me. Would you be willing to (request a doable) action? Spend a few minutes memorizing the sentences so you can use them naturally when needed.

With your partner, practice using Caspersen's Framework to address the scenario "in the moment." Take turns playing each role, using the framework.

### Narrative: The Case of the Scholar's Uncivil Behavior

Professor Blue is a brilliant scholar but a poor communicator. She often works from home, and when she comes to campus, her door is closed and she rarely interacts with others. Most of the time, this does not pose a problem, but when Professor Grey attempts to talk with Professor Blue about a research project on which they are collaborating, she is consistently unavailable. Professor Grey has tried repeatedly to make an appointment with Professor Blue, but she is not responding to calls, texts, or email messages. The research project is grant-funded, and the quarterly report is due. Finally, Professor Grey receives a return email from Professor Blue and is astonished to discover that the email is copied to the Dean and Director chastising Professor Grey and accusing her of sending harassing messages.

After your CR of Casperson's Framework, complete the following reflection questions:

- What was most challenging for you during this role-play exercise?

_____

_____

_____

_____

- What was most comfortable for you during this role-play exercise?

_____

_____

_____

_____

## 3. Paired Activity: The Caring Feedback Model

With your partner, review the six steps of the Caring Feedback Model. Using the following narrative, play the roles and practice using the model to resolve the conflict. Then switch roles and practice them again.

### Narrative: The Case of the Physician's Rude Behavior Pattern

Susan is the nurse manager of a bustling ICU and strives to foster excellent patient care among the members of her team. Dr. Nu is an experienced hospitalist with a reputation for being impatient with nurses, especially those newly hired or from the float pool. The unit is understaffed and extremely busy, so Julie, a registered nurse, has floated to the unit to help. Julie calls Dr. Nu about a patient concern. Dr. Nu interrupts, laughs, and says, "Is that all you called about? Is this a real nurse?" before listening further to understand the patient condition. Julie restates her concern, and once Dr. Nu understands, he orders the appropriate actions. Julie carries out the orders, and the patient situation improves. However, the exchange between Dr. Nu still troubled Julie. Later in the shift, Julie consults her charge nurse about the matter, who confirms that this is a pattern of behavior that other nurses on the unit tend to tolerate because Dr. Nu is respected for his excellent patient care. Julie decides to speak to the unit nurse manager, Susan, about Dr. Nu's behavior pattern and how it is harmful even though it has become an accepted practice. Susan agrees and decides to respond to Dr. Nu's behavior pattern using the Caring Feedback Model.

After your CR of the Caring Feedback Model, complete the following reflection questions:

- What was most challenging for you during this role-play exercise?

  _____

  _____

  _____

  _____

- What was most comfortable for you during this role-play exercise?

  _____

  _____

  _____

  _____

## 4. Paired Activity: Concerned, Uncomfortable, and Safety (CUS) Model

With your partner, review the three steps of the CUS Model. Using the following narrative, play the roles and practice using the model to resolve the conflict. Then switch roles and practice them again.

### Narrative: The Case of the Off-Going Nurse's Uncivil Handoff

Terry is a registered nurse who works at a busy cardiac unit at a large urban regional hospital. She cares for her mother living with Alzheimer's disease and has been experiencing difficulties arriving to places on time due to her role as a caretaker. She was late that morning to her shift at the cardiac unit, and Tia, the off-going nurse, provided her with the following handoff: "Geez, Terry, where have you been? You're late as usual. It's been a crazy, busy shift and I can't wait to get out of here. See if you can manage to get this information straight for once. You should know the patient in 204—you took care of her yesterday, so you should know what's going on. She was on 4S forever. Now she is our problem. She has a bunch of treatments that need to be done and medications that need to be given. You need to check her vital signs too—I've been way too busy to do them. So, that's it—I'm out of here. If I forgot something, it's not my problem. Just check the record."

After your CR of the CUS Model, complete the following reflection questions:

- What was most challenging for you during this role-play exercise?

_____

_____

_____

_____

- What was most comfortable for you during this role-play exercise?

_____

_____

_____

_____

## 5. Paired Activity: DESC Model

With your partner, review the four steps of the DESC Model. Using the following narrative, play the roles and practice using the model to resolve the conflict. Then switch roles and practice them again.

### Narrative: The Case of Co-Teaching in Nursing Education

Professor Brown, DNP, RN, is a part-time clinical lecturer in a college of nursing. She wears many hats both inside the college as a clinical lecturer and outside the college, as she is also a family nurse practitioner with a thriving practice. Professor Brown likes to keep on the cutting edge of science for her classes and thought it would be a fantastic idea to ask Professor Dimitri—a PhD-prepared, renowned content expert in their college—to co-facilitate a class with her. During class, however, Professor Dimitri interrupted several times to correct Professor Brown or add to her point, disrupting Professor Brown's train of thought. In the moment, Professor Brown felt diminished in front of the class after this incident but carried on through the duration of the class. Upon further reflection, Professor Brown decided that, even though the stakes were high and she wanted to maintain a good relationship with Professor Dimitri, it was important to address the situation in more detail and come to an agreement about how she would like to be treated in the future.

After your CR of the DESC Model, complete the following reflection questions:

- What was most challenging for you during this role-play exercise?

  _____

  _____

  _____

  _____

- What was most comfortable for you during this role-play exercise?

  _____

  _____

  _____

  _____

## 6. Paired Activity: PAAIL Method

With your partner, review the five steps of the PAAIL Method. Using the following narrative, play the roles and practice using the model to resolve the conflict. Then switch roles and practice them again.

### Narrative: The Case of the Nursing Student's Aggression About Clinical Placement

Mario is a senior level nursing student eagerly looking forward to his next clinical placement. He has requested placement in the Cardiac Intensive Care Unit (CICU). Mario expects his request to be accepted by his clinical instructor, Professor Taylor, because he has "the grades." Mario is very excited about the pending placement because he believes being assigned to the CICU will eventually lead to being accepted in a CRNA program. When assignments are made, Mario is placed on the orthopedic floor of a hospital several miles from his home. Mario is devastated and angry. He bursts into Professor Taylor's office angrily demanding to have his clinical placement changed to the CICU.

After your CR of the PAAIL Method, complete the following reflection questions:

- What was most challenging for you during this role-play exercise?

_____

_____

_____

_____

- What was most comfortable for you during this role-play exercise?

_____

_____

_____

_____

## 7. Group Activity: Share Uncivil Encounters and Create a Cognitive Rehearsal

As directed by your facilitator, follow these steps to create a group CR.

**Step 1:** After spending time learning about and applying various evidence-based frameworks using prewritten scenarios, participants assemble into small groups of five to six members. Each member should describe an uncivil encounter that has happened in their academic or work environment and share the encounter with their group.

**Step 2:** With your group, select one uncivil encounter from those shared within the group. Then select an evidence-based approach to "script" a response to address the uncivil encounter.

**Approach:**

_____

_____

_____

_____

**Script:**

_____

_____

_____

_____

**Step 3:** Members choose roles to act out the encounter and apply their "script." Group members not selected for the role-play will assume the role of observers.

**Step 4:** The facilitator oversees the role-play and facilitates a comprehensive coaching and debriefing session. Successful facilitator-led debriefing requires creating safe learning spaces for reflection to help identify aspects of the individual and team performance that went well, aspects that need improvement, and effective ways to address future situations. Some examples of debriefing questions include:

1.  For actors: What was it like to be part of this experience?

2.  For observers: What was it like to observe the experience?

3.  For all participants and observers:

    a.  How would you describe the experience?

    b.  What went well, and what would you do again?

    c.  What did you learn? How might you apply what you have learned in your clinical practice?

    d.  What might be done differently next time?

# Reflection

Take the _Clark Conflict Negotiation Challenge_ to improve your conflict negotiation skills and build relationships. To begin, consider a conflict you have experienced or are experiencing with a friend, family member, coworker, classmate, neighbor—or anyone you choose. Use the following steps to work through the conflict. Once you have completed the _Clark Conflict Negotiation Challenge_, consider sharing your observations with a trusted colleague, friend, or family member.

1.  Briefly describe the situation and identify the individual(s) involved.

    _____

    _____

    _____

    _____

2.  Highlight the key issues and perceived reason(s) for the conflict.

    _____

    _____

    _____

3.  If you addressed the situation, what strategies did you use? Were they effective?

    _____

    _____

    _____

4.  Describe how the conversation started, progressed, and ended.

    _____

    _____

    _____

5.  Upon reflection, how satisfied are you with the outcome? What are your next steps?

    _____

    _____

    _____

6.   If you avoided addressing the situation, what kept you from addressing it?

_____

_____

_____

_____

7.   Upon reflection, how satisfied are you with your decision not to address the situation?

_____

_____

_____

_____

## Reference

Maxfield, D., & Grenny, J. (2017). Crucial moments in healthcare: Patient safety and quality of care impacted by silence around five common workplace issues. *VitalSmarts*, 1–6.

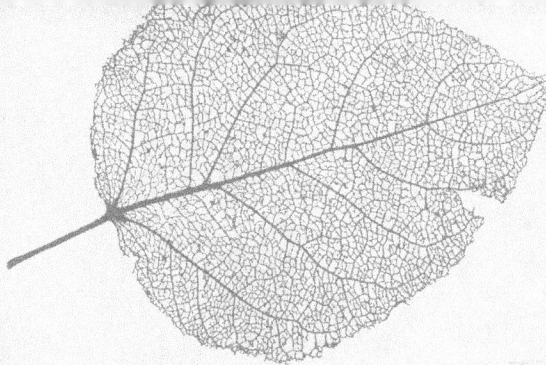

# 6

# The Power of Leadership, Visioning, and Finding Our WHY

### LEARNING OUTCOMES

- Describe characteristics of PEAK leaders.

- Identify Kouzes and Posner's Five Practices of Exemplary Leadership.

- Identify Kouzes and Posner's Ten Commitments of Exemplary Leadership.

- Create a personal, professional vision for the future related to nursing and healthcare.

- Craft an individual WHY statement that reflects your life purpose and the difference you wish to make in the world.

- Describe factors associated with an effective mentoring relationship.

# Key Concepts

After reading the chapter, test your understanding of the concepts with short answers.

1. Identify the four characteristics of a PEAK leader.

    _____

    _____

    _____

    _____

2. Define the four characteristics of a PEAK leader.

    _____

    _____

    _____

    _____

3. Identify the Five Practices of Exemplary Leadership according to Kouzes and Posner as referenced in Chapter 6.

    _____

    _____

    _____

    _____

4. Identify the Ten Commitments of Exemplary Leadership according to Kouzes and Posner as referenced in Chapter 6.

    1. _____

    2. _____

    3. _____

    4. _____

5. _____

6. _____

7. _____

8. _____

9. _____

10. _____

5. What are three important developmental activities discussed in Chapter 6 that can help one grow as a leader in nursing and healthcare?

_____

_____

_____

_____

6. According to the literature, identify three factors related to effective mentoring.

1. _____

2. _____

3. _____

# Rationale for Implementation

After reading the chapter, test your understanding of the concepts with short answers.

1. Why is it important to exemplify the characteristics of a PEAK leader in nursing and healthcare?

_____

_____

_____

_____

2. Why is it important to craft a personal, professional vision for the future?

_____

_____

_____

_____

3. Why is it important to find our individual WHY?

_____

_____

_____

_____

4. Why is it important to engage in mentorship and lifelong learning in nursing and healthcare?

_____

_____

_____

_____

# Application of the Concepts

Working with a partner, complete the following exercises as directed by your facilitator(s).

## 1. Paired Activity: Crafting a Personal, Professional Vision for the Future

As directed by your facilitator, take some time to answer the following questions, taking notes so you can remember your answers. Then pair up with a partner and share your answers. Finally, choose one take-away that the pair of you found most insightful and share that with the class.

1. How would I like others to describe me, my role, and my contributions in nursing and healthcare?

_____

_____

_____

_____

2. What legacy or indelible footprint do I aspire to leave during my career and upon retirement?

_____

_____

_____

_____

3. What aspects of my career bring me the most gratification and meaning?

_____

_____

_____

_____

## 2. Paired Activity: Creating and Sharing Your Individual WHY Statement

As directed by your facilitator, prior to the next learning session, spend some time thinking about question number one and developing an answer. Then complete the next step (number two). Bring your new WHY statement to class.

1. Using Sinek's template, create your individual WHY statement:

   TO (contribution)_____ SO THAT (impact)_____.

2. Share your individual WHY with a trusted friend, mentor, colleague, or family member.

3. With another colleague during an in-class learning session, discuss the following:

   - What did you learn from the process of creating a WHY statement?

   - What feedback did you receive about your WHY statement?

4. With the larger group, discuss the following question: What is the most important point you learned from creating an individual WHY statement and having it reviewed by a trusted friend, mentor, colleague, or family member?

## Reflection

It is important to periodically reflect and build upon your individual WHY statement since a well-developed WHY statement provides guidance and direction during turbulent times. One example of recent turbulence is the challenges faced during the COVID-19 pandemic. Keeping a thoughtful focus on your WHY can help sustain motivation to fulfill a larger purpose in nursing and healthcare. To continue to build your WHY statement, mark your calendar to revisit the following questions one to two months after completing this exercise. Share your answers with a trusted friend, family member, or colleague.

1. Revisit your WHY statement. Is there anything about your WHY statement you would like to change? Why or why not? If you revised your WHY statement, write it down.

_____

_____

_____

_____

2. What barriers do you perceive may impact your ability to achieve your WHY? How can these barriers be addressed?

_____

_____

_____

_____

3. What strengths do you have to achieve your WHY? Is there anything further you can do to bolster these strengths?

_____

_____

_____

_____

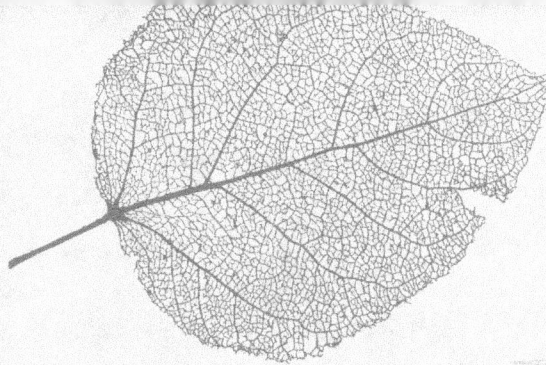

# 7

# Optimizing Self-Care and Professional Well-Being

## LEARNING OUTCOMES

- Describe the impact of stress and burnout in nursing and healthcare.

- Discuss the relationship between stress and incivility in nursing and healthcare.

- Identify contributors and outcomes to high stress in nursing practice and nursing education using the Conceptual Model for Fostering Civility in Nursing Education and the Conceptual Model for Fostering Civility in Nursing Education Adapted for Practice.

- Use the Personal Health Assessment to establish a baseline of personal well-being.

- Define change, transition, and the three stages an individual experiences during change according to the Bridges Transition Model.

- Identify at least three strategies to help manage external stress in nursing and healthcare that could affect individual well-being if left unaddressed.

- Discuss the role of resilience through mindfulness in managing stress.

- Implement at least one self-care exercise from Chapter 7 and evaluate its effectiveness.

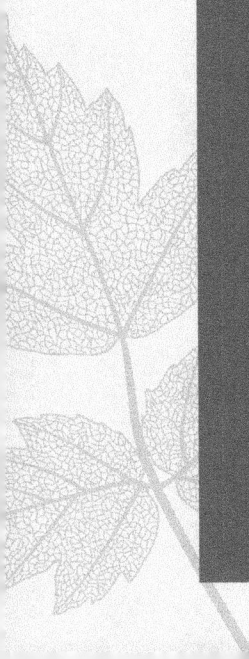

# Key Concepts

After reading the chapter, test your understanding of the concepts with short answers.

1. Describe the impact of stress in nursing and healthcare.

_____

_____

_____

_____

2. Define how stress relates to burnout.

_____

_____

_____

_____

3. How does stress relate to incivility in nursing and healthcare?

_____

_____

_____

_____

4. According to the Conceptual Model for Fostering Civility in Nursing Education Adapted for Practice, identify contributors to stress in nursing practice.

_____

_____

_____

_____

5. According to the Conceptual Model for Fostering Civility in Nursing Education, identify contributors to stress in nursing education.

_____

_____

_____

_____

6. Describe the meaning of change and transition according to Bridges and the three stages an individual experiences during change according to the Bridges Transition Model.

_____

_____

_____

_____

7. Identify the four health domains that can be measured using the Gourgouris and Apostolopoulos (2020) Personal Health Assessment.

_____

_____

_____

_____

8. Identify and describe at least three strategies to help manage external stress in nursing and healthcare.

_____

_____

_____

_____

9. Define resilience and mindfulness.

_____

_____

_____

_____

10. Identify habits to cultivate mindfulness to integrate into an everyday routine.

_____

_____

_____

_____

# Rationale for Implementation

After reading the chapter, test your understanding of the concepts with short answers.

1. Why is it important to manage stress in academic and practice settings?

_____

_____

_____

_____

2. Why is it important for individuals to assess their personal health?

_____

_____

_____

_____

3. During a stressful event, what happens to the brain at the biological level, and why is it important for sound cognition to manage stress?

_____

_____

_____

_____

# Application of the Concepts

Working independently and with a partner, complete the following exercises as directed by your facilitator(s).

## 1. Reflection and Sharing Activity: Creating Personal Positive Affirmations for Professional Development

1. Create a positive affirmation tailored to helping you grow as a professional in nursing or healthcare. One example could be, "I am letting go of negative thoughts. I will embrace opportunities to continue growing and developing as a professional." Write your positive affirmation down for the next steps.

_____

_____

_____

_____

2. Share your positive affirmation with a trusted colleague, friend, family member, or fellow learner. Discuss what makes this affirmation important to your professional development.

3. Then, take turns saying your positive affirmation out loud or silently in your mind.

4. Discuss how you felt after practicing saying your positive affirmation. Is there anything you would change about your positive affirmation? Why or why not?

_____

_____

_____

_____

## 2. Group Activity: Creating Expressions of Gratitude

As directed by your facilitator, take some time to answer the following questions, taking notes so you can remember your answers. Then pair up with a partner and share your answers and feedback. Finally, complete steps 5 and 6 to reflect and follow through with your expression of gratitude.

1.  Think about goals you have accomplished in the past month in your professional role as a nurse or healthcare professional, no matter how large or small. Did anyone help you along the way to accomplish your goals? Did you have access to resources to accomplish your goals that, if not present, would have otherwise made it much more difficult to achieve goals? Then, take notes about your accomplishments in the past month and people and resources who helped you achieve these accomplishments.

    _____

    _____

    _____

    _____

2.  Create a gratitude statement about people who helped you achieve your accomplishments, thanking them for their contributions.

    _____

    _____

    _____

    _____

3.  Take turns sharing your statement of gratitude with a small group of learners.

4.  How did you feel after sharing your gratitude statement? Offer feedback to other learners about their gratitude statements.

    _____

    _____

    _____

    _____

5. Since sharing your gratitude statement with a group of learners, is there anything you would change about your approach to creating and sharing a gratitude statement? Why or why not?

_____

_____

_____

_____

6. Share your gratitude statement with the person who helped you achieve your goals in an email or in person outside of the learning session.

_____

_____

_____

_____

## Reflection

Reflect upon the gratitude statements you created and how you felt after sharing your gratitude statements with the person for whom you are grateful.

1. Reflect about the response you received from the person for whom you were grateful. How did the other person respond? How did you feel after sharing your gratitude statement? If you were stressed before sharing this statement, how did you feel in terms of being stressed after you shared your gratitude statement?

_____

_____

_____

_____

2.  Since sharing your gratitude statement, is there anything you would like to change or add to your approach? Why or why not?

    _____

    _____

    _____

    _____

## Reference

Gourgouris, E., & Apostolopoulos, K. (2020). *7 keys to navigating a crisis: A practical guide to emotionally dealing with pandemics & other disasters*. The Happiness Center.

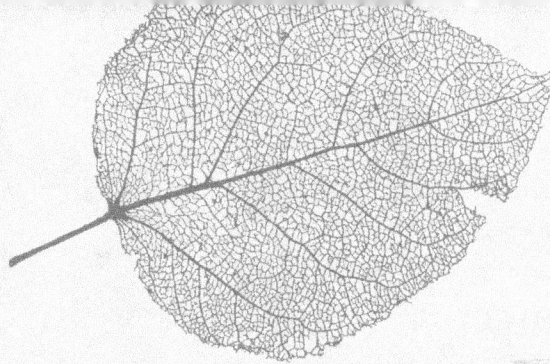

# 8

# Leadership Support and Raising Awareness for Organizational Change

### LEARNING OUTCOMES

- Define the Pathway for Fostering Organizational Civility (PFOC).

- Explain how organizational behavior informs the process of fostering organizational change for civility according to the PFOC.

- Illustrate the difference between buy-in and ownership in supporting change initiatives to foster organizational civility.

- Describe the role of organizational leadership in fostering civility and health work environments.

- Discuss how to enlist leadership support and raise awareness (Step 1 of the PFOC).

- Discuss strategies to assess the organizational culture (Step 2 of the PFOC).

# Key Concepts

After reading the chapter, test your understanding of the concepts with short answers.

1.  Define the Pathway for Fostering Organizational Civility (PFOC) and the first two steps of the PFOC.

    _____

    _____

    _____

    _____

2.  Describe unique aspects of organizational behavior that influence change and transformation.

    _____

    _____

    _____

    _____

3.  Explain the difference between *buy-in* and *ownership* in asking for support from organizational leaders about implementing a civility and health work environment initiative.

    _____

    _____

    _____

    _____

4.  Describe the importance of organizational leadership in fostering workplace civility.

    _____

    _____

    _____

    _____

5.  Discuss one method to enlist leadership support and raise awareness as Step 1 of the PFOC.

_____

_____

_____

_____

6.  Discuss strategies to assess the organizational culture as Step 2 of the PFOC.

_____

_____

_____

_____

## Rationale for Implementation

After reading the chapter, test your understanding of the concepts with short answers.

1.  Why is it important to gain the support of organizational leaders to implement civility and health work environment initiatives?

_____

_____

_____

_____

2.  Why is it important to assess the work environment using one of the organizational culture measurement tools provided in Chapter 8?

_____

_____

_____

_____

# Application of the Concepts

Working with a partner, complete the following exercises as directed by your facilitator(s).

## 1. Role-Play Activity: Using Role-Play to Practice Enlisting Leadership Support and Raising Awareness for Fostering Civility in the Workplace

1.  Using the information presented on pages 134 to 138 about civility in the workplace, harmful effects of incivility, benefits of civility, and civility in healthcare, create a brief script or bullet-pointed outline to act out (role-play) being an employee who secured a meeting with a high-level executive individual or team to advocate for organizational attention and resources to develop and implement a healthy work environment initiative.

_____

_____

_____

_____

### Example Template

- Brief introduction of the problem (i.e., workplace incivility), benefits of civility and healthy work environments
- Data points to illustrate the problem
- Proposed action and resources needed to foster healthy work environments

2.  Use the script to provide the person acting in the role of an executive with an overview of the problem, data to illustrate the problem, data to support benefits of civility, and proposed actions needed to foster healthy work environment. One learner will play the role of an executive listening, and the other will use their composed script.

3.  Once the script is delivered, ask your partner for feedback. Is there anything you would edit or add to the script? Why or why not?

_____

_____

_____

_____

Your facilitator may direct you to repeat the role play by taking opposite roles from before. The facilitator may also ask you to share your experiences and insight with the class.

## 2. **Paired Activity:** Comparing and Contrasting Tools to Assess the Organizational Culture

There are six different assessment tools introduced in Chapter 8 to assess the health of an organization's culture and work environment. Pair up with a colleague and review the following six assessment tools described on pages 139 to 142 of Chapter 8 and/or conduct an internet search to explore other relevant assessment tools including assessment tools being used in your workplace:

- American Association of Critical-Care Nurses (AACN) Healthy Work Environment Tool
- Workplace Incivility/Civility Survey
- Workplace Relational Civility Scale
- Civility, Respect, Engagement in the Workforce Scale
- Negative Acts Questionnaire – Revised
- Healthy Work Environment Inventory

1. Considering these tools, which one would you select to measure the health and work environment of your organization? Discuss the reasoning for your selection.

   _____

   _____

   _____

   _____

2. Were there multiple tools that could be useful for assessing the health of the work environment at your organization? If so, please describe the other tools that could be used, and the reasoning for these thoughts.

   _____

   _____

   _____

   _____

# Reflection

Enlisting leadership support is a first step to assessing the organizational culture to foster a healthier work environment. Reflect on the script you practiced in the role play to introduce facts and reasons to assess and foster healthier work environments. Next, consider how the tool you selected in Activity #2 might be integrated into your script and presentation to the executive leadership individual or team.

1.  How did you feel while acting in the role of an employee speaking to a high-level executive team or individual about the extent to which workplace incivility is a problem and the importance of healthy work environments? Is there anything you would have changed about your script? Why or why not?

    _____

    _____

    _____

    _____

2.  Likewise, how did you feel while acting in the role of a high-level executive listening to an employee about the extent to which workplace incivility is a problem and the importance of fostering healthy work environments? What are your thoughts about having a neutral party administer an evidence-based assessment tool to measure the organizational culture? Is there anything you would suggest the other learner to change in their script? Why or why not?

    _____

    _____

    _____

    _____

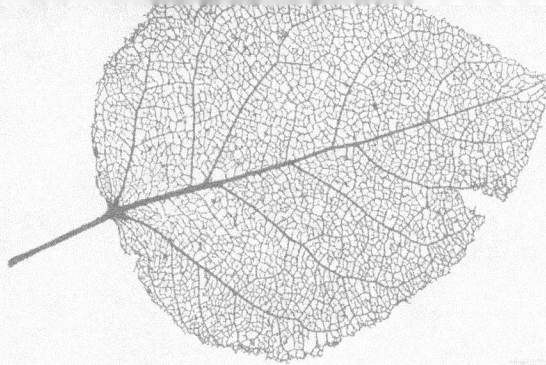

# 9

# Galvanizing a High-Performing Civility Team

## LEARNING OUTCOMES

- Specify characteristics of high performing teams in nursing and healthcare.

- Describe psychological safety as a part of nursing and healthcare team norms.

- Define a Civility Team and state its primary two-fold purpose.

- Identify and describe cultural factors within organizational cultures.

- Discuss how a Civility Team or designee can utilize information gleaned from the organizational assessment to foster a healthy work environment.

- Describe a golden moment in your time working on nursing and/or healthcare teams and how it informs your perspectives about your current work situation.

# Key Concepts

After reading the chapter, test your understanding of the concepts with short answers.

1. Define and describe a *team*.

   _____

   _____

   _____

   _____

2. Describe characteristics of high-performing teams.

   _____

   _____

   _____

   _____

3. Describe psychological safety.

   _____

   _____

   _____

   _____

4. Identify, define, and describe cultural factors to examine as part of a Civility Team's organizational assessment.

   _____

   _____

   _____

   _____

5.  List the two primary overall functions of Civility Teams.

_____

_____

_____

_____

6.  Identify other important functions of the Civility Team.

_____

_____

_____

_____

# Rationale for Implementation

After reading the chapter, test your understanding of the concepts with short answers.

1.  Why is it important to assemble a Civility Team of diverse membership and backgrounds?

_____

_____

_____

_____

2.  Why is psychological safety a key element of fostering high-performing teams in nursing and healthcare?

_____

_____

_____

_____

# Application of the Concepts

Working with a partner, complete the following exercises as directed by your facilitator(s).

## 1. Group Activity: Creating a Concept Map for High-Performing Teams

1. For this activity, assemble into groups of four to five members and place the major concept of high-performing teams in the center of the map. Then build and connect sub-concepts and related ideas to show interrelationships with the major concept of high-performing teams. Following is an example template of a concept map with sub-concepts and related ideas.

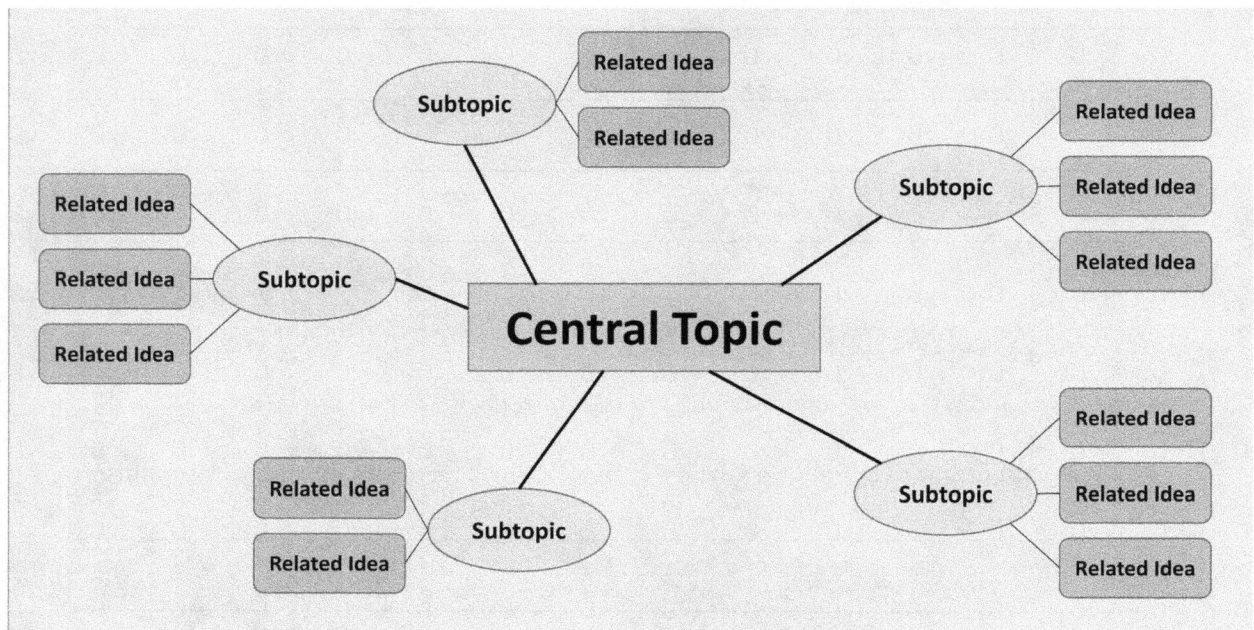

2. Once the concept map is completed, each group should share their map with one or two other groups to discuss similarities and differences.

## 2. Group Activity: Assessing Psychological Safety in Work Teams

1. After assembling into groups, reread pages 152–153 of the text.

2. Reflect upon a group, team, or committee in which you are currently or most recently a member.

3. Discuss in small groups the seven questions posed by Edmondson (2019, p. 20) listed here as they relate to the group, team, or committee identified in question #2.

    1. If you make a mistake on this team, it is often held against you.

    2. Members of this team are able to bring up problems and tough issues.

3. People on this team sometimes reject others for being different.

4. It is safe to take a risk on this team.

5. It is difficult to ask other members of this team for help.

6. No one on this team would deliberately act in a way that undermines my efforts.

7. Working with members of this team, my unique skills and talents are valued and utilized.

Once you have had an opportunity to discuss these seven questions, a spokesperson from each group will share a "gem" or a "pearl of wisdom" with the larger group.

## Reflection

The author defines a *golden moment* as a zestful, dynamic time in our working life when we felt inspired, validated, and filled with a sense of well-being, joy, and delight. Living a golden moment means we are experiencing the incredible joy and satisfaction of being part of a high-performing team engaged in very challenging, yet rewarding and meaningful work. Reflect on your career and respond to the following questions:

1. Have you ever experienced a golden moment in your career? Think back to a time (or perhaps it is now in your current workplace) when being a member of a team or committee left you feeling joyful, zestful, and positively unstoppable.

   _____

   _____

   _____

   _____

2. What was the experience like? How would you describe it?

   _____

   _____

   _____

   _____

3.  Rate your golden moment on a scale ranging from 0 to 10 (0 = absolute worst work experience ever to 10 = most incredible work experience ever). If it is truly a golden moment your rating will be 9 or 10/10!

_____

_____

_____

_____

4.  As you reflect on your current work situation, if your rating is less than 7 or 8, or even lower, examine whether your current work setting is the right fit for you.

_____

_____

_____

_____

# Reference

Edmondson, A. C. (2019). *The fearless organization: Creating psychological safety in the workplace for learning, innovation, and growth*. John Wiley & Sons.

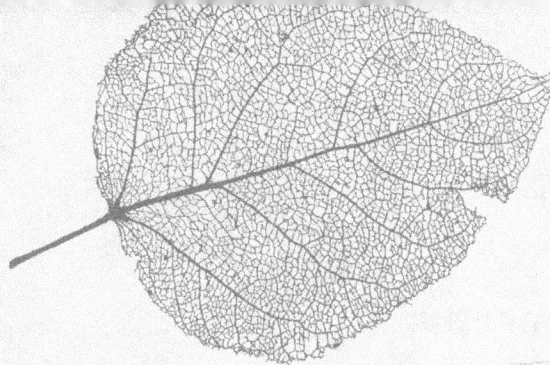

# 10

# Develop, Implement, and Evaluate a Data-Driven Action Plan

## LEARNING OUTCOMES

- Identify John Kotter's (1996) elements for creating an organizational vision statement as part of designing a data-driven action plan (Step 4 of the PFOC) to promote organizational civility.

- Discuss the importance of crafting a compelling civility vision statement.

- Define the meaning and purpose of co-creating a Civility Charter and team norms.

- Understand the role of accountability in fulfilling team norms.

- Identify the steps to implement the data-driven action plan (Step 5 of the PFOC).

- Discuss the process for evaluating the data-driven action plan (Step 6 of the PFOC).

# Key Concepts

After reading the chapter, test your understanding of the concepts with short answers.

1. List the six elements needed for an organizational vision statement according to Kotter (1996).

    _____

    _____

    _____

    _____

2. List the eight steps to Latham's (1995) framework to create an organizational vision statement.

    _____

    _____

    _____

    _____

3. Define a *Civility Charter* and its purpose.

    _____

    _____

    _____

    _____

4. Define the meaning of *team norms*.

    _____

    _____

    _____

    _____

5. Define *accountability*.

_____

_____

_____

_____

6. Define and explain the purpose of *shared governance* in practice and in education.

_____

_____

_____

_____

7. As part of a Civility Education Plan, what are the three types of workshops the Civility Team could facilitate to foster a shared understanding and motivation for achieving greater organizational civility?

_____

_____

_____

_____

8. What steps are included in a data-driven action plan? (Step 5 of the PFOC)

_____

_____

_____

_____

9.  What does an evaluation plan include for the data-driven action plan? (Step 6 of the PFOC)

_____

_____

_____

_____

# Rationale for Implementation

After reading the chapter, test your understanding of the concepts with short answers.

1.  Why is it important to create a comprehensive and compelling vision statement?

_____

_____

_____

_____

2.  Why is it important to co-create and maintain team norms and a Civility Charter?

_____

_____

_____

_____

3.  Why is accountability important to upholding team norms?

_____

_____

_____

_____

# Application of the Concepts

Working with a small group, complete the following exercises as directed by your facilitator(s).

## 1. Group Activity: Creating a Civility Vision Statement

In small groups of four to five members, each member should briefly summarize their organizational statements. After all members have had an opportunity to describe their organizational statements, the group will select an organization among learners to use for creating a Civility Vision Statement. Review the selected organization's mission, vision, and values, and take 20 minutes to brainstorm about crafting a vision statement using the following formula:

---

### Vision Statement Formula

The vision (purpose) of the civility and healthy workplace initiative is to _____ for (target population) _____ to fulfill the purpose of _____.

---

Upon completion of this statement, identify specific strategies to share the civility vision with other members of the organization. Share the statement and communication strategies with the larger group. Include at least one key takeaway point from this exercise that could help future efforts to create a Civility Vision Statement.

## 2. Group Activity: Co-Creating Team Norms

In small groups of four to five members, co-create a list of team norms that are relevant to the organization's vision, mission, values, and commitment to its members. A spokesperson from each small group will share their answers to the following questions with the larger group of learners.

1. Share team norms created with the larger group.

   _____

   _____

   _____

   _____

2.  Discuss why the team norms created are important for the organization.

_____

_____

_____

_____

3.  Describe strategies for how members of the organization could be held accountable to upholding these team norms.

_____

_____

_____

_____

## Reflection

Based on the experiences from the prior activities, reflect on the process of creating team norms for an organization in small groups. Then answer the following questions:

1.  Was the experience of creating norms as you expected? Why or why not?

_____

_____

_____

2.  Is there anything different you would do in the future when creating team norms? Describe what these actions would be if so.

_____

_____

_____

_____

# References

Kotter, J. P. (1996). *Leading change*. Harvard Business Review Press.

Latham, J. R. (1995, April). Visioning: The concept, trilogy, and process. *Quality Progress, 28*(4), 65–68.

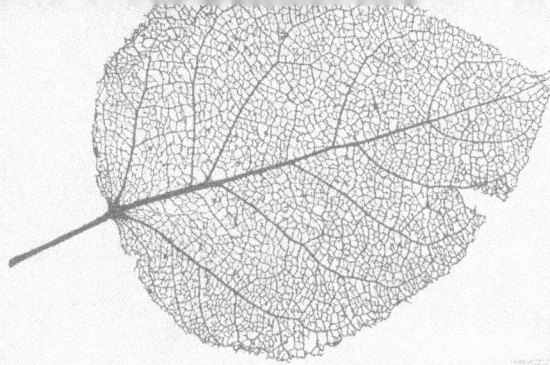

# 11

# Securing Civility Into the Organizational Culture Through Policy Development

### LEARNING OUTCOMES

- Explain the overall goal of a healthy work environment policy as a fundamental feature to shape and maintain a civil organizational culture.

- Discuss key factors to develop an effective policy to embed civility and healthy work environments into the organizational culture (Step 7 of the PFOC).

- Define and discuss the SMART policy to address and report incivility and to reward civility.

- Identify and discuss steps in the decision-making model for managing issues related to incivility.

- Describe the importance of using civility metrics to gauge employee performance and to use for hiring decisions.

# Key Concepts

After reading the chapter, test your understanding of the concepts with short answers.

1.  Describe the overall goal of a healthy work environment policy.

    _____

    _____

    _____

    _____

2.  Describe the key factors for effective policy development.

    _____

    _____

    _____

    _____

3.  Identify and describe the five elements of the SMART policy.

    _____

    _____

    _____

    _____

4.  Describe steps one could take to address and manage a report of uncivil behavior in the workplace.

    _____

    _____

    _____

    _____

5. Identify and describe the steps of the decision-making model for managing issues related to incivility.

_____

_____

_____

_____

6. List some questions interviewees could ask job applicants about issues of diversity, equity, and inclusion as related to civility.

_____

_____

_____

_____

# Rationale for Implementation

After reading the chapter, test your understanding of the concepts with short answers.

1. Why is it important to create a healthy work environment policy?

_____

_____

_____

_____

2. Why is it important to hire for civility and link civility to performance metrics?

_____

_____

_____

_____

# Application of the Concepts

Working with a small group, complete the following exercises as directed by your facilitator(s).

## 1. Group Activity: Healthy Work Environment Policy Critique

Reread the healthy work environment policy exemplar on pages 195 to 199. Then, gather into small groups to critique the policy using the questions listed below. Identify items or content you might add, delete, or modify when considering a healthy work environment policy for the specific organization. After critiquing the policy, re-convene as a larger group and share at least three key takeaways from your small group discussion.

**Policy critique:** Using a scale from 1-4 (1 = strongly disagree, 2 = disagree, 3 = agree, 4 = strongly agree), rate the level of agreement for the following questions. Then discuss your ratings and rationale within your small group.

1.  To what extent does the policy meet the overall objective of creating and sustaining a healthy work environment to transform the organizational culture?

    _____

    _____

    _____

    _____

2.  To what extent are the policy purpose, policy statement, and commitment to civility well defined and clearly stated for all members of the organization?

    _____

    _____

    _____

    _____

3. To what extent are the list of shared values and statement on incivility and other workplace aggressions relevant to fostering a healthy work environment?

_____

_____

_____

_____

4. To what extent are the examples of incivility and other workplace aggressions and the examples of desired behaviors relevant to fostering a healthy work environment?

_____

_____

_____

_____

5. To what extent are the procedure and reporting statements clearly stated for all members of the organization?

_____

_____

_____

_____

6. To what extent does the policy promote systemic change and long-term sustainability?

_____

_____

_____

_____

## 2 Group Activity: Civility Conversation Role-Play Between Manager and Reported Employee

Assemble into small groups and identify a real or potential uncivil scenario that could occur in your workplace. Read pages 202 to 203 ("Civility Conversations for Managers and Supervisors") to write a script based on the scenario. The script includes the role of a "manager" and the role of an "employee" who will be meeting to discuss a complaint that has been filed against the employee accusing them of a serious act of workplace aggression. Your group will identify group members to play the roles of "manager" and "employee." After completing the script of the uncivil encounter, the actors will role-play the scenario for the larger group.

Facilitator-led debriefing questions:

1. **For actors:** What was it like to be part of this experience? What thoughts and/or feelings were evoked?

2. **For observers:** What was it like to observe the experience? What did you see? What did you hear?

3. **For all** participants and observers:

   a. How would you describe the conversation?

   b. What went well, and what would you do again?

   c. What was most effective about the conversation?

   d. What might be done differently next time?

   e. How might you apply what you have learned in your clinical practice?

## Reflection

Reflect on whether your specific organization has implemented a policy to foster civility and a healthy work environment. Then answer the following questions:

1. Does a healthy work environment policy exist?

   _____

   _____

   _____

   _____

2.  If so, does it include a confidential, step-by-step procedure to serve as a road map for reporting both acts of civility and incivility?

_____

_____

_____

_____

3.  Does the policy reflect a commitment to diversity, equity, and inclusion?

_____

_____

_____

_____

4.  Is the policy easily accessible and widely disseminated?

_____

_____

_____

_____

5.  If a healthy work environment policy does not exist in your organization, what steps might you take to assemble and lead a team to develop and implement a healthy work environment policy?

_____

_____

_____

_____

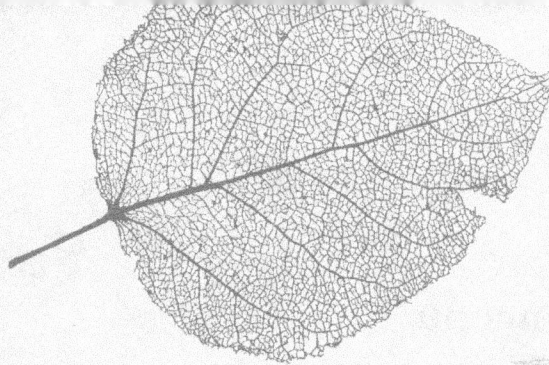

# 12

# Celebrating Civility: A Powerful Engine to Uplift and Transform the Profession

## LEARNING OUTCOMES

- Identify methods to consolidate gains and build momentum as part of Step 8 of the PFOC.

- Describe methods to expand the civility initiative and sustain organizational transformation as part of Step 8 of the PFOC.

- Discuss the importance of celebrating civility in an organization of nursing and healthcare professionals.

- Explain the importance of hope and optimism to transform nursing and healthcare professions.

# Key Concepts

After reading the chapter, test your understanding of the concepts with short answers.

1.  Identify methods to consolidate gains and build momentum as part of Step 8 of the PFOC.

    _____

    _____

    _____

    _____

2.  Discuss processes to expand the civility initiative as a part of sustaining organizational transformation for a healthier, more civil work environment.

    _____

    _____

    _____

    _____

3.  What is *tragic optimism*, and why is it important to informing hope and optimism to transform health professions?

    _____

    _____

    _____

    _____

4.  What is *toxic positivity*, and why is it important to avoid during efforts to foster hope and optimism to transform health professions?

    _____

    _____

    _____

    _____

## Rationale for Implementation

After reading the chapter, test your understanding of the concepts with short answers.

1. Why is it important to celebrate civility in an organization?

_____

_____

_____

_____

2. Why is it important to expand the civility initiative?

_____

_____

_____

_____

## Application of the Concepts

Working with a small group, complete the following exercises as directed by your facilitator(s).

### 1. Research & Group Activity: Celebrating Civility: A Tiered Approach

Conduct an independent internet search of ways to celebrate or reward civility in the workplace and identify at least one civility celebration or reward for three cost levels: no cost, low cost, and higher cost. Then, share your findings with a small group of other learners. Using the following prompts, evaluate ideas for celebrating civility at each cost level in a small group, and discuss strategies to integrate the celebration or reward into the work or learning environment.

1. For each cost tier (no cost, low cost, and higher cost), evaluate the pros and cons for designing and implementing the civility celebration ideas found through an internet search.

2. Select the top idea for each cost tier to share with a larger group of learners.

3. Describe the rationale for selecting each idea considering the cost tier and the main motivation for these selections.

4. Discuss the most appealing aspects about celebration ideas found at the three cost levels.

5. Discuss how you would advocate for enacting these ideas in your workplace.

## 2. Case Study Group Activity: Navigating and Sustaining Interest in the Civility Initiative

As directed by the facilitator, read the following scenario, and then gather in small groups to discuss it using the questions that follow as prompts.

### Scenario

For the past year, Professor Gomez has been a major contributor for the School of Nursing's Civility Team. As a founding member of the Civility Team, Professor Gomez has invested significant time and effort to ensure its success. The Civility Team's progress has been substantial, with several notable accomplishments, including completing a baseline comprehensive assessment and plan for creating and sustaining a civil work environment, the development and implementation of an organizational civility policy to address uncivil behavior, and the development and implementation of a web-based confidential reporting system for tracking and addressing uncivil incidents. Professor Gomez implemented a pre-post survey to measure and document the effect of the Civility Team's interventions and found that, overall, faculty and staff morale about promoting a civil environment has improved as correlated to the Civility Team's efforts. Although Professor Gomez has been a strong contributing member of the Civility Team, she is concerned that her recently funded research project will require her to devote more time and effort to research and less time to Civility Team responsibilities. Professor Gomez has a strong desire for the Civility Team to succeed and for their efforts to remain a priority in the School of Nursing. When Professor Gomez communicates her need to redirect her focus to research, she discovers that another Civility Team member has similar competing demands. As the team problem-solves the situation, they realize that a process is needed to expand the civility initiative and bring new members onto the Civility Team in an ongoing manner.

1. How could Professor Gomez best communicate her needs to the Civility Team in a manner that is respectful to the team and to herself?

   _____

   _____

   _____

   _____

2. What processes could be put in place to monitor and reward time spent on the Civility Team as part of the organization's vision to create and sustain a healthy work environment?

   _____

   _____

   _____

   _____

3. In addition to time, what other resources may be needed to expand the civility initiative?

_____

_____

_____

_____

4. How might the organizational bylaws assist in bringing new members on the Civility Team?

_____

_____

_____

_____

## Reflection

Stories engage and activate emotion and connect us to one another. Telling a simple, powerful, relevant story breathes life and relevance into everyday life. When we share stories, we make meaning of and provide context for understanding our own and others' lived experiences. For this reflection exercise, begin by rereading the quote on page 223 of the text: "We are writing history right now, and we hold the pen. We are and can be the heroes in this story!" Take 10 to 15 minutes to compose a story from your life or work experience that sheds a positive light on how navigating and overcoming challenges can lead to a positive and productive future.

_____

_____

_____

_____

_____

_____

_____

_____

www.ingramcontent.com/pod-product-compliance
Lightning Source LLC
Chambersburg PA
CBHW072000220326
41599CB00034BA/7067